Complete Diet & Health Management Workbook

Dr. Arthur H. Kebo

Complete Diet & Health Management Workbook

ISBN-13: 978-1477487389
ISBN-10: 1477487387

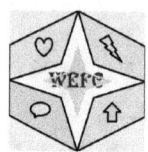

Book Website:

> https://www.createspace.com/3881369

WordPress Blog Website:

> http://twelvefoundations.wordpress.com/

Twitter Website:

> https://twitter.com/#!/twelvefoundatio

Facebook Website:

> http://www.facebook.com/arthurkebo

Printed in the United States of America

Table of Contents

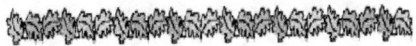

Preface

Health is one of the greatest assets that we have, and our children and family are another of our greatest assets, and we have a responsibility to take care of their health. Without health, we cannot work or play or live. Therefore, it is imperative that we maintain our optimal health, at all times. This being said, it is not always the easiest thing to do. In order to assist you, this workbook was developed to manage your day-to-day health. Often, without a solid health maintenance plan, it is our tendency to become slack or indifferent to our health regime. Our usual lifestyle and busyness sets in, and our health takes a back seat. It is when we become sick or incapacitated that we realize how we had neglected to maintain our health, and only wish we had kept some type of management program.

This workbook is designed to help you keep a record of your health on a daily basis, so that you can analyze your progress every month. Without this record, it is very difficult to see that progress; and without seeing progress, it is hard to keep yourself motivated to maintain the proper health plan. This indifference to your health drags on month to month, then year to year, until you find yourself in the hospital or taking extended time away from work, or even losing your job. Even if you do not lose your job, health affects your performance at work, which in turn affects promotions and salaries and career plans. It not only affects your work performance, but at the same time, it affects your family and your general personality.

If you are always tired, due to all the toxins that have accumulated in your body, which is stored in your fat cells, this will affect your mood, and consequently, your relationship with others. Moreover, these toxins in your body create an environment which is a breeding ground for bacteria, viruses, parasites and cancer cells. It is paramount that you eat a lot of healthy food, such as vegetables and fruits, which helps your body to fight these invaders; exercise properly to circulate nutrients and oxygen to your cells, and flush toxins out of your body that create illnesses; and avoid things such as stress and tobacco and sugar which act negatively to your health. The author has tried to provide this worksheet at minimal cost, in order to save you thousands of dollars in medical costs, later.

It is the author's wish that through the use of this complete diet and health maintenance workbook, you will be able to keep a daily tab on such things as your calories, cholesterol level, blood pressure, nutrition plan, relaxation plan, exercise plan, etc.; and not only maintain your health, but to improve your health through successful dieting and a concrete exercise plan. The worksheets in this book are designed to approach your health management from all possible angles that contribute to your well-being. It is small enough to carry in your pocket, at all times—easily accessible to you at the fitness club, restaurant, while jogging, and at work.

A healthy person is a happy person. Let us start today, and not delay a day longer: one day of delay becomes a month of delay, and a month a year. This is the day to take that commitment to stay healthy, avoid the hospital and that exorbitant medical bill, and live to see your grandchildren grow up. It starts now. Or, send this workbook to your grandparents or your father for his Father's Day gift. It will probably be the most important gift that you can give them—your care.

Overall Health Measure Graph

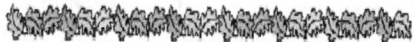

From the data recorded on the worksheets for each health category in this workbook, enter the health level you calculated below on the graph:

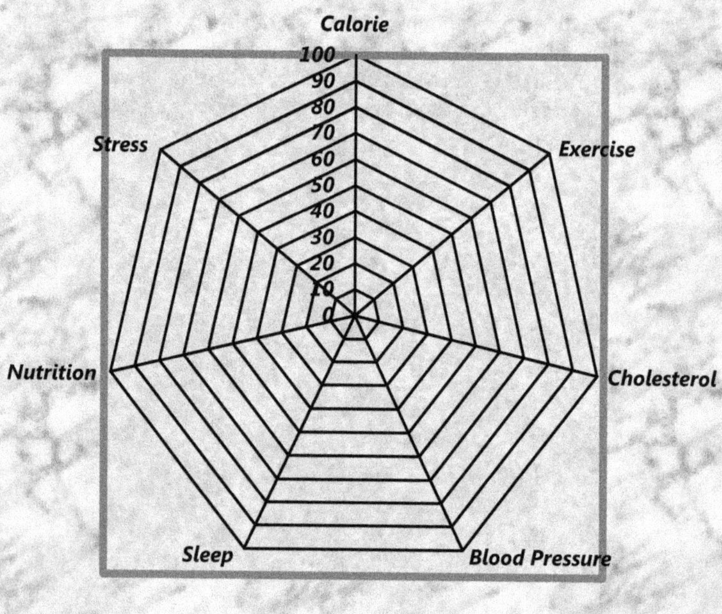

Calorie
Stress
Exercise
Nutrition
Cholesterol
Sleep
Blood Pressure

100
90
80
70
60
50
40
30
20
10
0

This is the visual presentation of your overall health management this month to give you an idea of your general condition. It is to provide you guidance on what areas you are doing well, and what areas you need to improve, next month. Use the information to discuss your health plan with your fitness/health professional.

Daily Calorie Intake & Calorie Use Comparison Sheet

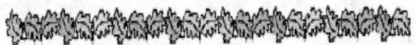

Enter below, the calorie intake from page 9 and the estimated calorie use from exercises, jogging, and daily metabolism based on such things as body size and job type from page 16. Next, subtract the Calorie Use amount from the Calorie Intake amount for each day, and enter the differences in the right column:

DAY	CALORIE INTAKE	CALORIE USE	DIFFERENCE
1	+	−	=
2	+	−	=
3	+	−	=
4	+	−	=
5	+	−	=
6	+	−	=
7	+	−	=
8	+	−	=
9	+	−	=
10	+	−	=
11	+	−	=
12	+	−	=
13	+	−	=
14	+	−	=
15	+	−	=
16	+	−	=
17	+	−	=
18	+	−	=
19	+	−	=
20	+	−	=
21	+	−	=
22	+	−	=
23	+	−	=

24	+		−		=	
25	+		−		=	
26	+		−		=	
27	+		−		=	
28	+		−		=	
29	+		−		=	
30	+		−		=	
31	+		−		=	

Add the Difference Subtotals in the right column, and enter the result below:

MONTHLY CALORIE DIFFERENCE TOTAL	=

Divide the Monthly Calorie Difference Total above with the number of days in the month:

DIVIDE BY THE NUMBER OF DAYS IN THE MONTH	÷ 30 or 31

Enter the result below:

NUMBER OF CALORIES OVER/UNDER PER DAY	=

If the Number Of Calories Over/Under Per Day is a negative number, you are under the daily calorie intake, so you may increase your calorie, unless you are on a diet program. If your Number of Calories Over/Under Per Day is a positive number, you are over the daily calorie intake, so you need to decrease the amount of calories you eat by that amount every day.

On the graph on page 6, enter the score from 0 to 100 for your calories category. For every 10 calories you are over or under per day, subtract 1 point from the calorie score of 100.

Meal Calorie Record Sheet

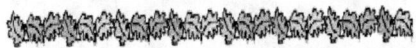

Enter the calories for each meal every day. Look at the Meal/Food Product Sample Calorie Amount Table on pages 14 and 15 for approximate calorie amounts:

DAY	BREAK FAST	LUNCH	DINNER	SNACK	DAILY SUBTOTAL
1					=
2					=
3					=
4					=
5					=
6					=
7					=
8					=
9					=
10					=
11					=
12					=
13					=
14					=
15					=
16					=
17					=
18					=
19					=
20					=
21					=
22					=
23					=
24					=
25					=
26					=

27					=
28					=
29					=
30					=
31					=

Meal Calorie Monthly Calculation Worksheet

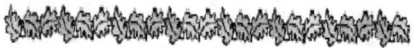

Add the Daily Subtotals in the right column, and enter the result below:

MONTHLY CALORIE INTAKE TOTAL	=

Divide the Monthly Calorie Intake Total above by the number of days in the month:

DIVIDE BY THE NUMBER OF DAYS IN THE MONTH	÷ 30 OR 31

Enter the result below:

AVERAGE DAILY CALORIE CONSUMPTION	=

This is your average calorie consumption every day. It is important to analyze the amount of calories you use every day, and adjust your calorie consumption to match the calorie use.

Meal Calorie Monthly Monitoring Graph

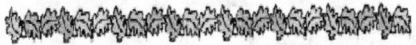

Add the Breakfast, Lunch, Dinner and Snack columns, and enter their totals below:

TOTAL MONTHLY BREAKFAST CALORIES	TOTAL MONTHLY LUNCH CALORIES	TOTAL MONTHLY DINNER CALORIES	TOTAL MONTHLY SNACK CALORIES

Divide these Monthly Totals above by the number of days in the month:

DIVIDE BY THE NUMBER OF DAYS IN THE MONTH	÷ 30 or 31 DAYS

Enter the results below:

AVERAGE DAILY BREAKFAST CALORIES	AVERAGE DAILY LUNCH CALORIES	AVERAGE DAILY DINNER CALORIES	AVERAGE DAILY SNACK CALORIES

Multiply the Average Daily Calories for each meal above by 100. Then, divide that result by the Average Daily Calorie Consumption from page 10, in order to find out the Percentage of Daily Calories for each meal category.

(Average Daily Meal Calories x 100) ÷ Average Daily Calorie Consumption = Percentage of Daily Calories

or

$$\frac{Average\ Daily\ Meal\ Calories}{Average\ Daily\ Calorie\ Consumption} = \frac{Percentage\ of\ Daily\ Calories}{100\%}$$

Enter your results below:

Breakfast

$$\frac{Calories}{Calories} = \frac{\%}{100\%}$$

11

<u>**Lunch**</u>

$$\frac{\text{Calories}}{\text{Calories}} = \frac{\text{_____ \%}}{100\%}$$

<u>**Dinner**</u>

$$\frac{\text{Calories}}{\text{Calories}} = \frac{\text{_____ \%}}{100\%}$$

<u>**Snack**</u>

$$\frac{\text{Calories}}{\text{Calories}} = \frac{\text{_____ \%}}{100\%}$$

Graph the Percentage of Daily Calories for each type of meal (breakfast, lunch, dinner, snack) above on the Meal Calorie Monthly Analysis Graph below, in order to give you a visual overview of your overall calorie intake per meal.

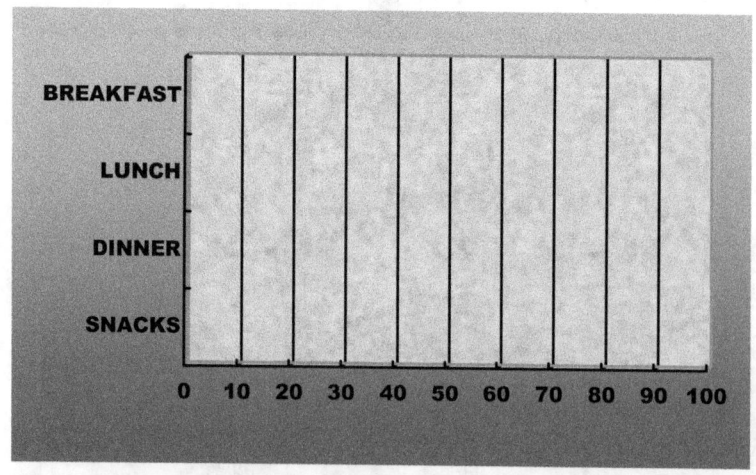

For optimal health, it is advisable to eat a larger breakfast and smaller dinner, since your calorie usage and physical activity decreases at night, unless you exercise after dinner. It is also advisable to minimize the calories taken from snacks, if you find from the graph that the majority of your calories are taken from the snacks, instead of the three regular meals. It is important to eat a good, balanced breakfast, since it will give you energy for your day's activities, and provide energy for your brain to work effectively.

Meal/Food Product Sample Calorie Amount Table

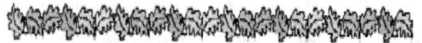

PROTEINS	CALORIES
Steak (100g)	200 ~ 250
Roasted Chicken (100g)	200 ~ 350
Smoked Salmon (100g)	100 ~ 200
Egg (1 large)	80 ~ 100
Tofu (100g)	60 ~ 80

CARBOHYDRATES	CALORIES
Wheat Bread (1 slice)	60 ~ 70
Baked Potato	100 ~ 120
White Rice (1 cup)	180 ~ 210
Baked Beans (1 cup)	200 ~ 400
Pasta (1 cup)	210 ~ 240

VEGETABLES	CALORIES
Lettuce (100g)	10 ~ 20
Tomato	25 ~ 35
Cucumber	40 ~ 50
Spinach (1 cup)	5 ~ 10
Onion	50 ~ 70

FRUITS	CALORIES
Apple	100 ~ 120
Orange	70 ~ 100
Grapes (1 cup)	50 ~ 100
Raisins (1 cup)	450 ~ 550
Banana	90 ~ 120

DESSERTS	CALORIES
Apple Pie (1 slice)	250 ~ 350
Chocolate Cake (100g)	450 ~ 550
Donut	100 ~ 130
Chocolate Pudding (100g)	350 ~ 400
Vanilla Ice Cream (100g)	200 ~ 300

DRINKS	CALORIES
Coffee	3 ~ 5
Orange Juice (1 cup)	100 ~ 130
Soda (1 can)	150 ~ 250
Milk (1 cup)	130 ~ 150
Tea	3 ~ 5

SNACKS	CALORIES
Cheddar Cheese (1 cup)	500 ~ 550
Potato Chips (100g)	500 ~ 600
Candy Bar	200 ~ 300
Plain Popcorn (1 cup)	30 ~ 50
Brownie (1 square)	200 ~ 250

Daily Activities Calorie Use Record Sheet

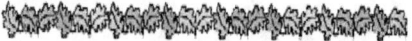

Calculate your approximate daily calorie usage using the table on page 18, and record your calorie usage amount below:

DAY	ACTIVITIES DESCRIPTION	CALORIES
1		
2		
3		
4		
5		
6		
7		
8		
9		
10		
11		
12		
13		
14		
15		
16		
17		
18		
19		
20		
21		
22		
23		
24		
25		
26		
27		

28		
29		
30		
31		

Monthly Calorie Use Calculation Worksheet

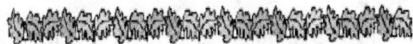

Add the Daily Activity Calorie Use Subtotals in the right column, and enter the result below:

APPROXIMATE MONTHLY CALORIE USE TOTAL	=

Divide the Approximate Monthly Calorie Use Total above by the number of days in the month:

DIVIDE BY THE NUMBER OF DAYS IN THE MONTH	÷ 30 OR 31

Enter the result below:

AVERAGE DAILY CALORIE USE	=

This is your average calorie use every day. Depending on your weight loss program, you will need to adjust this amount, accordingly.

On the graph on page 6, enter your score between 0 and 100 for your exercise category. For each day you exercised at least 30 minutes, add 3.33 points for a 30-day month and 3.23 for a 31-day month.

Activity Sample Calorie Use Amount Table

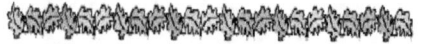

EXERCISE TYPE	APPROXIMATE CALORIE USE
Walking (3 mph / 10 minutes)	35 ~ 40
Cycling (10 ~ 15 mph / 10 minutes)	90 ~ 100
Aerobics (10 minutes)	50 ~ 80
Freestyle Swimming (10 minutes)	90 ~ 110
Weight Lifting (10 minutes)	30 ~ 40
Basketball (10 minutes)	80 ~ 100
Cleaning (10 minutes)	30 ~ 40
Electrical Work (10 minutes)	30 ~ 40
Sitting (10 minutes)	20 ~ 30
Construction Work (10 minutes)	40 ~ 60
Car Maintenance (10 minutes)	30 ~ 40
Child-Rearing (10 minutes)	30 ~ 40
Playing (10 minutes)	35 ~ 45
Cooking (10 minutes)	20 ~ 30
Hard Labor (10 minutes)	80 ~ 90
Farm & Ranch Work (10 minutes)	70 ~ 80
Jogging (10 minutes)	70 ~ 80
Running (8 mph / 10 minutes)	140 ~ 160
Yard Cleaning (10 minutes)	40 ~ 50
Jump Rope (10 minutes)	100 ~ 120
Handball (10 minutes)	130 ~ 140
Golf (10 minutes)	30 ~ 40
Carpentry (10 minutes)	35 ~ 45
Lawn Mowing (10 minutes)	50 ~ 60
Playing Guitar (10 minutes)	20 ~ 30
Rock Climbing (10 minutes)	120 ~ 130
Stretching & Balance (10 minutes)	30 ~ 40
Daily Calorie Usage Without Exercise (Just simple work and play.)	2,000 (average person)

Daily Jogging Record Sheet

DAY	DISTANCE	APPROXIMATE CALORIES BURNED FROM JOGGING
1		
2		
3		
4		
5		
6		
7		
8		
9		
10		
11		
12		
13		
14		
15		
16		
17		
18		
19		
20		
21		
22		
23		
24		
25		
26		
27		
28		

29		
30		
31		

Add the daily Approximate Calories Burned From Jogging Subtotals in the right column, and enter the result below:

APPROXIMATE MONTHLY CALORIES BURNED FROM JOGGING	=

Divide the Approximate Monthly Calorie Burned From Jogging amount above by the number of days in the month:

DIVIDE BY THE NUMBER OF DAYS IN THE MONTH	$\div$ 30 OR 31

Enter the result below:

AVERAGE DAILY CALORIE BURNED FROM JOGGING	=

This is your average calorie burned from jogging every day. Depending on your weight loss program, you will need to adjust this amount, accordingly. Walking, jogging or swimming is all good calorie burners, so it is good to do them at least three times a week or every day, if possible, in moderation. Keep your blood pressure, heart condition and pulse monitored.

Cholesterol Record Sheet

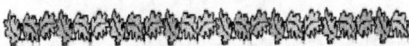

Monitor and enter your cholesterol levels for each category below, at certain times throughout the year:

LDL	HDL	TRIGLYCERIDE	TOTAL CHOLESTEROL

Cholesterol Monitoring Graph

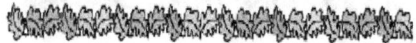

Plot your cholesterol level on the graphs below to give you an idea whether your cholesterol level is stationary, rising, or falling, and take corrective actions, as necessary:

LDL

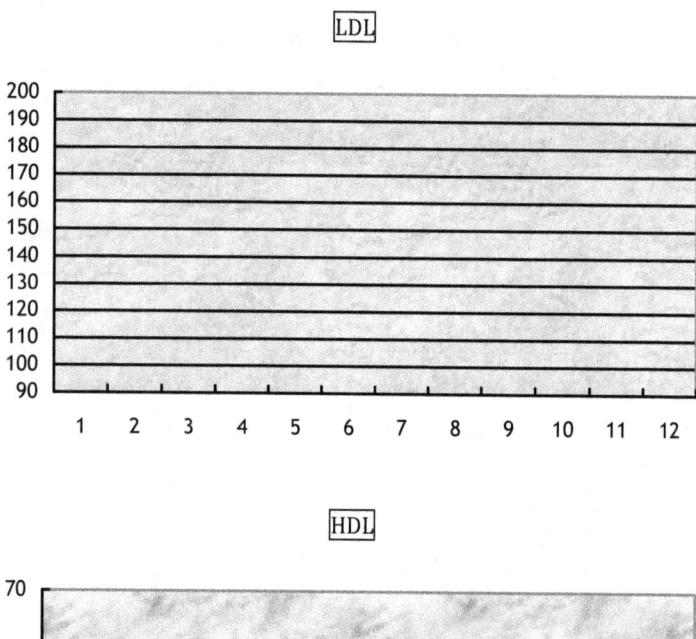

HDL

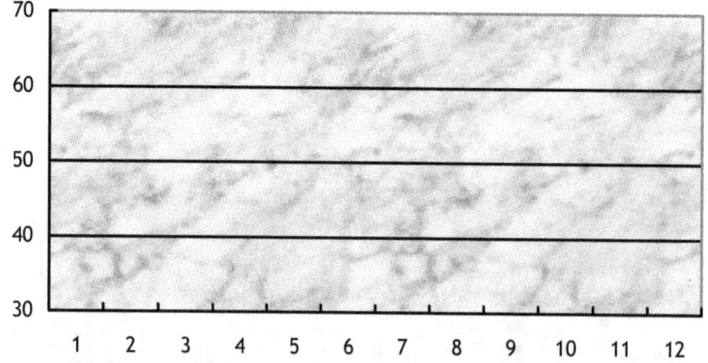

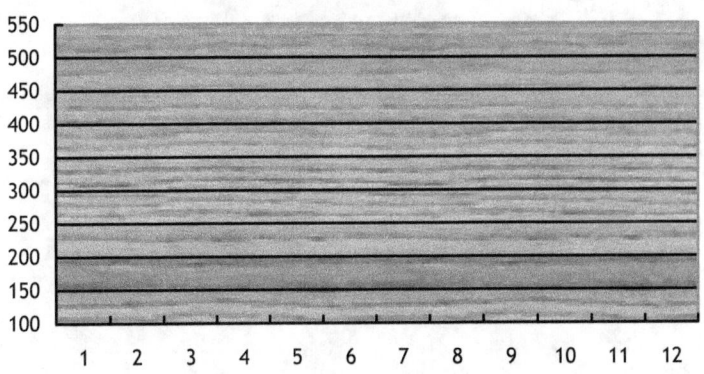

TRYGLYCERIDE

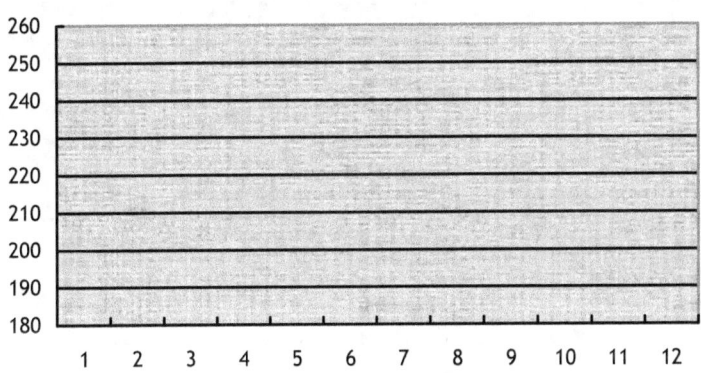

TOTAL CHOLESTEROL

On the graph on page 6, enter your score between 0 and 100 for your cholesterol category. If your cholesterol level is very good, give yourself a score between 80 to 100; if your cholesterol level needs improvement, give yourself a score between 40 to 70; and if your cholesterol level is not so good, give yourself a score between 10 to 30.

Blood Pressure Record Sheet

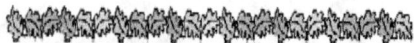

Monitor and enter your daily blood pressure levels for each category below:

DAY	SYSTOLIC	DIASTOLIC
1		
2		
3		
4		
5		
6		
7		
8		
9		
10		
11		
12		
13		
14		
15		
16		
17		
18		
19		
20		
21		
22		
23		
24		
25		
26		
27		
28		

29		
30		
31		

Blood Pressure Monitoring Graph

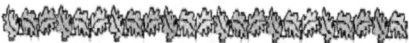

Plot your blood pressure level on the graphs below to give you an idea whether your blood pressure level is stationary, rising, or falling, and take corrective actions, as necessary:

SYSTOLIC

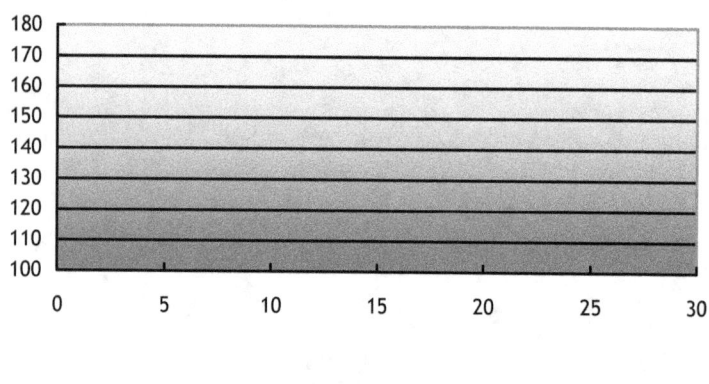

DIASTOLIC

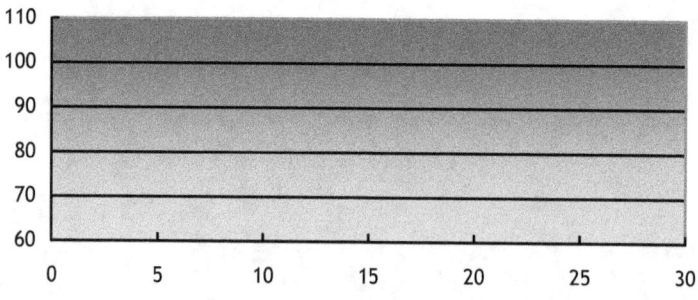

On the graph on page 6, enter your score between 0 and 100 for your blood pressure category. If your blood pressure level is very good, give yourself a score between 80 to 100; if your blood pressure level needs improvement, give yourself a score between 40 to 70; and if your blood pressure level is not so good, give yourself a score between 10 to 30.

Sleep Hour Record Sheet

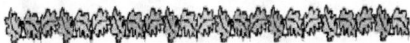

Enter the time you fell asleep, the time you woke up, and the total hours of sleep you got every day:

DAY	TIME FELL ASLEEP	TIME WOKE UP	TOTAL HOURS
1			
2			
3			
4			
5			
6			
7			
8			
9			
10			
11			
12			
13			
14			
15			
16			
17			
18			
19			
20			
21			
22			
23			
24			
25			
26			
27			

28			
29			
30			
31			

Sleep Cycle Calculation Worksheet

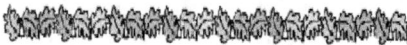

Add the Total Hours in the right column, and enter the result below:

MONTHLY SLEEP HOURS TOTAL	=

Divide the Monthly Sleep Hours Total above by the number of days in the month:

DIVIDE BY THE NUMBER OF DAYS IN THE MONTH	÷ 30 OR 31

Enter the Average Daily Sleep Hours amount below:

AVERAGE DAILY SLEEP HOURS	=

Divide the Average Daily Sleep Hours above by 90 minutes:

DIVIDE BY 90 MINUTES	÷ 90

Enter the result below:

DAILY AVERAGE COMPLETE SLEEP CYCLES	

The amount of sleep that a person needs depends on the individual, as well as other factors, such as age. On average, most adults needs around 7 to 9 hours of sleep every night, and a lot more if you are younger. Quality of sleep is also very important. On the graph on page 6, enter your score between 0 and 100 for your sleep category. If you feel you are getting a good night's sleep, give yourself a score between 80 to 100; if you feel that your sleep can improve, give yourself a score between 40 to 70; and if you feel that you are having a sleep disorder, give yourself a score between 10 to 30.

Sleeping Tips For Deep REM Sleep

1. Try to avoid food, alcohol, cigarettes or caffeinated drinks late at night.
2. Keep a record of your sleep hours, and know what your sleep patterns are.
3. Instead of struggling to fall asleep at a certain time, make a habit of waking up at the same time every morning; and then, your body will adjust to the hours.
4. Flood your body with light when you wake up by opening your curtains; and make the room dark when you sleep for deeper REM sleep.
5. Do not to deprive yourself of sleep every night, and try to catch up on lost sleep on the weekends, but keep a normal cycle of at least 7 hours of sleep every night throughout the week.
6. Do not do strenuous exercise or work before going to sleep.
7. Avoid sleeping during the daytime.
8. Walk and get proper exercise during the day.
9. Forget about work or worries during bedtime.
10. Do not work on a bright screen computer until bedtime.
11. Get a bed and pillow that matches your needs.
12. Drink herbal tea or listen to soft music and not loud music, in order to relax before sleeping.

Nutrition Record Sheet

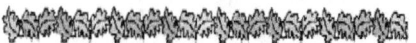

Keep a record of a few typical meals you regularly have throughout the month. Analyze them to see if you and your kids are getting the proper nutrition, and adjust your meal plans, depending on the findings, and as necessary. Below, are some tools to help you keep a record of your sample meals, and compare them with your government health agency's recommended daily nutrition amount, or what your health professional advises. You may take a look at the nutrition label on your food product to get a general idea of its nutritional content.

BREAKFAST #1 (Date: ___ / ___ / ___)

List the food items:

_____
_____
_____
_____

NUTRITIENT	ESTIMATED AMOUNT FOR THIS MEAL	YOUR GOVERNMENT OR HEALTH PROFESSIONAL'S RECOMMENDED DAILY AMOUNT
Calories		
Protein		
Carbohydrate		
Fat		
Saturated Fatty Acids		
Cholesterol		
Fiber		
Sodium		
Potassium		
Vitamin A		
Thiamin		

Riboflavin		
Niacin		
Vitamin B6		
Vitamin B12		
Vitamin C		
Vitamin D		
Vitamin E		
Vitamin K		
Calcium		
Iron		
(List Your Own)		
(List Your Own)		
(List Your Own)		
(List Your Own)		
(List Your Own)		

BREAKFAST #2 (Date: ___ / ___ / ___)

List the food items:

_____

_____

_____

_____

NUTRITIENT	ESTIMATED AMOUNT FOR THIS MEAL	YOUR GOVERNMENT OR HEALTH PROFESSIONAL'S RECOMMENDED DAILY AMOUNT
Calories		
Protein		
Carbohydrate		
Fat		
Saturated Fatty Acids		
Cholesterol		

Fiber		
Sodium		
Potassium		
Vitamin A		
Thiamin		
Riboflavin		
Niacin		
Vitamin B6		
Vitamin B12		
Vitamin C		
Vitamin D		
Vitamin E		
Vitamin K		
Calcium		
Iron		
(List Your Own)		
(List Your Own)		
(List Your Own)		
(List Your Own)		
(List Your Own)		

BREAKFAST #3 (Date: ___ / ___ / ___)

List the food items:

_____

_____

_____

_____

NUTRITIENT	ESTIMATED AMOUNT FOR THIS MEAL	YOUR GOVERNMENT OR HEALTH PROFESSIONAL'S RECOMMENDED DAILY AMOUNT
Calories		

Protein		
Carbohydrate		
Fat		
Saturated Fatty Acids		
Cholesterol		
Fiber		
Sodium		
Potassium		
Vitamin A		
Thiamin		
Riboflavin		
Niacin		
Vitamin B6		
Vitamin B12		
Vitamin C		
Vitamin D		
Vitamin E		
Vitamin K		
Calcium		
Iron		
(List Your Own)		
(List Your Own)		
(List Your Own)		
(List Your Own)		
(List Your Own)		

LUNCH #1 (Date: ___ / ___ / ___)

List the food items:

_____

_____

_____

_____

NUTRITIENT	ESTIMATED AMOUNT FOR THIS MEAL	YOUR GOVERNMENT OR HEALTH PROFESSIONAL'S RECOMMENDED DAILY AMOUNT
Calories		
Protein		
Carbohydrate		
Fat		
Saturated Fatty Acids		
Cholesterol		
Fiber		
Sodium		
Potassium		
Vitamin A		
Thiamin		
Riboflavin		
Niacin		
Vitamin B6		
Vitamin B12		
Vitamin C		
Vitamin D		
Vitamin E		
Vitamin K		
Calcium		
Iron		
(List Your Own)		
(List Your Own)		
(List Your Own)		
(List Your Own)		
(List Your Own)		

LUNCH #2 (Date: ___ / ___ / ___)

List the food items:

_____
_____
_____
_____

NUTRITIENT	ESTIMATED AMOUNT FOR THIS MEAL	YOUR GOVERNMENT OR HEALTH PROFESSIONAL'S RECOMMENDED DAILY AMOUNT
Calories		
Protein		
Carbohydrate		
Fat		
Saturated Fatty Acids		
Cholesterol		
Fiber		
Sodium		
Potassium		
Vitamin A		
Thiamin		
Riboflavin		
Niacin		
Vitamin B6		
Vitamin B12		
Vitamin C		
Vitamin D		
Vitamin E		
Vitamin K		
Calcium		
Iron		

(List Your Own)		
(List Your Own)		
(List Your Own)		
(List Your Own)		

LUNCH #3 (Date: ___ / ___ / ___)

List the food items:

_____

_____

_____

_____

NUTRITIENT	ESTIMATED AMOUNT FOR THIS MEAL	YOUR GOVERNMENT OR HEALTH PROFESSIONAL'S RECOMMENDED DAILY AMOUNT
Calories		
Protein		
Carbohydrate		
Fat		
Saturated Fatty Acids		
Cholesterol		
Fiber		
Sodium		
Potassium		
Vitamin A		
Thiamin		
Riboflavin		
Niacin		
Vitamin B6		
Vitamin B12		
Vitamin C		
Vitamin D		

	ESTIMATED AMOUNT FOR THIS MEAL	YOUR GOVERNMENT OR HEALTH PROFESSIONAL'S RECOMMENDED DAILY AMOUNT
Vitamin E		
Vitamin K		
Calcium		
Iron		
(List Your Own)		
(List Your Own)		
(List Your Own)		
(List Your Own)		
(List Your Own)		

DINNER #1 (Date: ____ / ____ / ____)

List the food items:

_____

_____

_____

_____

NUTRITIENT	ESTIMATED AMOUNT FOR THIS MEAL	YOUR GOVERNMENT OR HEALTH PROFESSIONAL'S RECOMMENDED DAILY AMOUNT
Calories		
Protein		
Carbohydrate		
Fat		
Saturated Fatty Acids		
Cholesterol		
Fiber		
Sodium		
Potassium		
Vitamin A		
Thiamin		
Riboflavin		

Niacin		
Vitamin B6		
Vitamin B12		
Vitamin C		
Vitamin D		
Vitamin E		
Vitamin K		
Calcium		
Iron		
(List Your Own)		
(List Your Own)		
(List Your Own)		
(List Your Own)		
(List Your Own)		

DINNER #2 (Date: ___ / ___ / ___)

List the food items:

_____

_____

_____

_____

NUTRITIENT	ESTIMATED AMOUNT FOR THIS MEAL	YOUR GOVERNMENT OR HEALTH PROFESSIONAL'S RECOMMENDED DAILY AMOUNT
Calories		
Protein		
Carbohydrate		
Fat		
Saturated Fatty Acids		
Cholesterol		
Fiber		

Sodium		
Potassium		
Vitamin A		
Thiamin		
Riboflavin		
Niacin		
Vitamin B6		
Vitamin B12		
Vitamin C		
Vitamin D		
Vitamin E		
Vitamin K		
Calcium		
Iron		
(List Your Own)		
(List Your Own)		
(List Your Own)		
(List Your Own)		
(List Your Own)		

DINNER #3 (Date: ___ / ___ / ___)

List the food items:

_____

_____

_____

_____

NUTRITIENT	ESTIMATED AMOUNT FOR THIS MEAL	YOUR GOVERNMENT OR HEALTH PROFESSIONAL'S RECOMMENDED DAILY AMOUNT
Calories		
Protein		

Carbohydrate		
Fat		
Saturated Fatty Acids		
Cholesterol		
Fiber		
Sodium		
Potassium		
Vitamin A		
Thiamin		
Riboflavin		
Niacin		
Vitamin B6		
Vitamin B12		
Vitamin C		
Vitamin D		
Vitamin E		
Vitamin K		
Calcium		
Iron		
(List Your Own)		
(List Your Own)		
(List Your Own)		
(List Your Own)		
(List Your Own)		

Note: There are other nutrients based on your specific needs, and food groups such as vegetables contain healthy chemicals to protect your body and boost immune systems. Likewise, some food items may not agree with your body. Each person should consult a health professional to design a diet that fits his or her needs and age, and strive to meet them every day.

Nutrition Calculation Worksheet

Add the total amount for each nutrient category above, and divide them by the number of meals you investigated. Then, enter the result in the far right column for each nutrient category. This is your Average Nutrient Per Meal that you are getting:

NUTRIENT	TOTAL AMOUNT	DIVIDED BY THE NUMBER OF MEALS	AVERAGE NUTRIENT PER MEAL
Calories		÷	=
Protein		÷	=
Carbohydrate		÷	=
Fat		÷	=
Saturated Fatty Acids		÷	=
Cholesterol		÷	=
Fiber		÷	=
Sodium		÷	=
Potassium		÷	=
Vitamin A		÷	=
Thiamin		÷	=
Riboflavin		÷	=
Niacin		÷	=
Vitamin B6		÷	=
Vitamin B12		÷	=
Vitamin C		÷	=
Vitamin D		÷	=
Vitamin E		÷	=
Vitamin K		÷	=
Calcium		÷	=
Iron		÷	=
		÷	=

(List Your Own)		÷	=
(List Your Own)		÷	=
(List Your Own)		÷	=
(List Your Own)		÷	=

Subtract your government health agency's recommended daily nutrition amount, or what your health professional advises, from the Average Nutrient Per Meal for each nutrient category:

NUTRIENT	AVERAGE NUTRIENT PER MEAL	SUBTRACT RECOMMENDED DAILY NUTRITION AMOUNT	DIFFERENCE LACKING OR EXCEEDING RECOMMENDED AMOUNT
Calories		—	=
Protein		—	=
Carbohydrate		—	=
Fat		—	=
Saturated Fatty Acids		—	=
Cholesterol		—	=
Fiber		—	=
Sodium		—	=
Potassium		—	=
Vitamin A		—	=
Thiamin		—	=
Riboflavin		—	=
Niacin		—	=
Vitamin B6		—	=
Vitamin B12		—	=
Vitamin C		—	=
Vitamin D		—	=
Vitamin E		—	=
Vitamin K		—	=
Calcium		—	=

Iron		$-$		$=$	
(List Your Own)		$-$		$=$	
(List Your Own)		$-$		$=$	
(List Your Own)		$-$		$=$	
(List Your Own)		$-$		$=$	
(List Your Own)		$-$		$=$	

If the amount is a positive number, you are exceeding the nutritional amount for each nutrient category compared to that of your government health agency's recommended daily nutrition amount, or what your health professional advises. If the amount is a negative number, you are lacking the nutritional amount for each nutrient category compared to that of your government health agency's recommended daily nutrition amount, or what your health professional advises.

Multiply the Average Nutrient Per Meal amount by 100 for each nutrient category. Then, divide that result by the Recommended Nutrition Amount, in order to find out the Percentage Actually Taken for each nutrient category. Enter the Percentage Actually Taken for each nutrient category on the Nutrition Monitoring Graph on the next page.

(Average Nutrient Per Meal x 100) ÷ Recommended Nutrition Amount = Percentage Actually Taken

or

$$\frac{Average\ Nutrient\ Per\ Meal}{Recommended\ Nutrition\ Amount} = \frac{Percentage\ Actually\ Taken}{100\%}$$

Nutrition Monitoring Graph

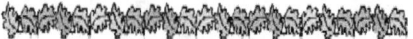

Enter the amount of the Percentage Actually Taken for each of the nutrient category from the previous page below:

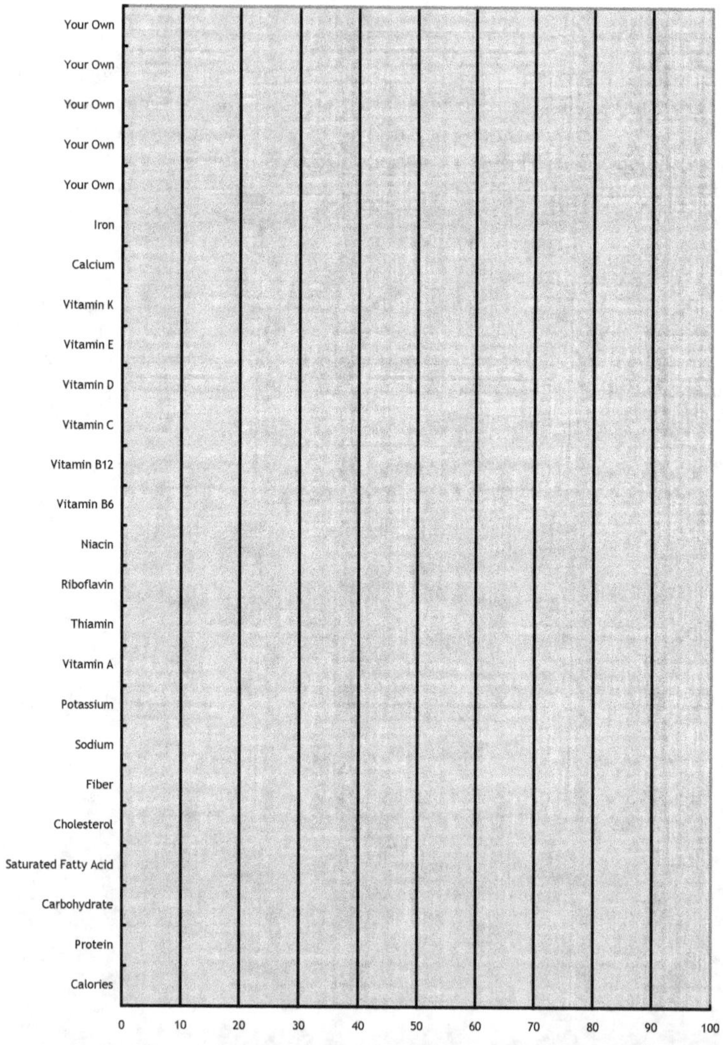

	0	10	20	30	40	50	60	70	80	90	100
Your Own											
Your Own											
Your Own											
Your Own											
Your Own											
Iron											
Calcium											
Vitamin K											
Vitamin E											
Vitamin D											
Vitamin C											
Vitamin B12											
Vitamin B6											
Niacin											
Riboflavin											
Thiamin											
Vitamin A											
Potassium											
Sodium											
Fiber											
Cholesterol											
Saturated Fatty Acid											
Carbohydrate											
Protein											
Calories											

On the graph on page 6, enter your score between 0 and 100 for your nutrition category. If you feel you are getting a proper nutrient intake, give yourself a score between 80 to 100; if you feel that your nutrient intake can improve, give yourself a score between 40 to 70; and if you feel that you are not getting your proper nutrient intake, give yourself a score between 10 to 30.

Stress Reduction Planning Sheet

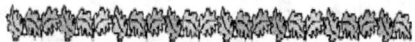

Enter the type of relaxation activity you had throughout the month below. Record the level of effectiveness for each activity you tested for future analysis:

DAY	ACTIVITY	MINUTES	SCORE (1 TO 100)
1			
2			
3			
4			
5			
6			
7			
8			
9			
10			
11			
12			
13			
14			
15			
16			
17			
18			
19			
20			
21			
22			
23			
24			
25			
26			

27			
28			
29			
30			
31			

List the five highest scoring relaxation activity you experienced. This will vary between different individuals. Try to focus on these activities, which you find are the most effective for you:

ORDER OF EFFECTIVENESS	ACTIVITY	SCORE
1		
2		
3		
4		
5		

Stress Prevention Action Plan

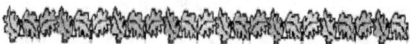

Not only is it important to relieve stress, but it is also important to reduce and prevent stress. List below, five things that you can do to reduce or prevent stress, such as making a priority list of things to do for the day, or delegating your work to your subordinates, or only taking important phone calls, etc. Try to apply them every day into your lifestyle:

PREVENTIVE MEASURES	DESCRIPTION

Relaxation – Suggested Methods

1. Manage your time better by prioritizing, scheduling, and monitoring your time.
2. Decide to eliminate things that take up your time, which are unnecessary or not as important.
3. Be able to say, "No."
4. Avoid individuals who are confrontational or argumentative.
5. Stop being a perfectionist and always demanding perfect standards where such standards are not required.
6. Avoid bitterness, and learn to forget.
7. Exercise every day to relieve stress.
8. Find a friend who you can share concerns, and who can relate to your circumstances, and give you helpful direction.
9. Do not try to do everything by yourself, but learn to delegate.
10. Set aside personal time for yourself.
11. Think positively, and do not be a pessimist.
12. Get a proper nutrition of vitamins and minerals, especially calcium.
13. Stop drinking, smoking, driving, or other things that may strain your heart.
14. Strive to do something you enjoy, at least once a day.
15. Get a pet.
16. Try aromatherapy, reading a book, listening to music, or getting a message—whatever works for you the best.
17. Learn to put your work aside from your mind, once you get home.
18. Learn to control your temper and blood pressure.
19. Step back, and learn to look at things from a different perspective.
20. Take a vacation ever-so-often, or change the environment.
21. Learn to do one thing at a time.
22. Plan well in ahead.
23. Get enough sleep.
24. Get a light snack, so you are not hungry.
25. Move to a country and culture where life is more enjoyable and slow-paced, rather than a country and culture where everything is busy and fast-paced.
26. Read one of this author's books on comedy.

Mental / Emotional Health Test

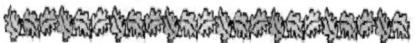

Enter your score truthfully, for each of the following questions, based on the following answers:

1. Strongly Disagree
2. Disagree
3. Somewhat Agree
4. Agree
5. Strongly Agree

	QUESTION	SCORE
1	Do you always feel pressured for time, and do not feel you have enough time?	
2	Do you feel yourself always irritated at situations or other people?	
3	Are you dissatisfied at yourself, or discouraged?	
4	Do you have any loss of appetite or insomnia or other physical signs of stress?	
5	Do you always feel tired, and have a lack of motivation?	
6	Do you find yourself drinking, or smoking, or eating excessively?	
7	Do you feel overwhelmed quite often by the things around you?	
7	Do you find yourself having less concentration and less ability to retain memory?	
8	Do you see any emotional swings in your behavior?	
9	Do you find yourself always dwelling on the negative things?	
10	Do you find that your mind is always on things that may happen, or problems at home or work?	
11	Do you feel that you are being taken advantage of?	
12	Are you unsure about your future?	
13	Do you find yourself always storing your emotions away without sharing them?	
14	Do you feel you are not getting enough sleep or rest?	

15	Do you find yourself dwelling on the past a lot?	
16	Do you feel that there is no place to vent your frustrations or release your stress?	
17	Do you feel that there are unreasonable demands placed upon your life?	
18	Are you having any relationship problems?	
19	Do you find yourself micromanaging or trying to do several things at once?	
20	Have you lost room for any humor or find yourself not laughing as much?	

Add the scores on the right column, and enter the result below:

TOTAL	=

Divide the Total above by the number of questions:

DIVIDE BY THE NUMBER OF QUESTIONS	÷ 20

Enter the result below to get your average score:

AVERAGE SCORE	=

The higher the average score, the higher possibility that you may have greater stress than you were aware of or was willing to admit. You need to find remedies now, before it may affect your overall health or family or work. May this serve as a wake-up call.

On the graph on page 6, enter your score between 0 and 100 for your stress management category. If you feel you are managing your stress effectively, give yourself a score between 80 to 100; if you feel that your stress management can improve, give yourself a score between 40 to 70; and if you feel that you are not managing your stress effectively, give yourself a score between 10 to 30.

Words Of Advice

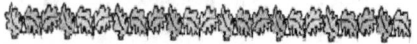

The secret to successfully maintaining your health is perseverance. You have to continue to monitor your health, not only in a general sense, but in all areas of your lifestyle. By diligently keeping a record of your activities and health performance, you will be able to identify areas you are lagging behind, and need to step up. Just like any business enterprise or military campaign, your body and mind needs careful attention, just as much as your car that you always wax, tune, fuel up and check. A sloppy management of your health results in a mediocre health, and eventual breakdown in one or more areas.

Most people make a New Year's resolution to exercise daily or cut back on calories and fatty food this year, but it never gets implemented or they stop following through with their determination. It is because they do not monitor it every day, and keep a detailed record. When you see the record on paper, then it motivates you to continue to maintain the record, and it gives you a goal to shoot for, in terms of real numbers. When you see the improvement over the month, it motivates you to continue. Without seeing that improvement every day on paper, the health management often becomes neglected over time. This is why New Year's resolutions for dieting and exercising never materialize.

It is important that you carry this workbook with you, and keep a record of your meals and exercise. When you visually observe the slimmer waist or greater energy at work, then you actually experience the thrill of your successful health management. It is too late when you end up in the hospital. Our body is complex, but it is also very simple: if you maintain it, it will take care of you. However, if you neglect it, it will fail you. Where your busyness, indifference and lack of motivation acts as obstacles to increasing your life span and leading a vibrant, happy life, this workbook will help to wage war against those negative forces working against you, and assist you in your commitment to healthy living. Live young, keep young, feel young, and continue to look young.

Other Books By The Author

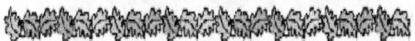

Home Economics: Budgeting & Expense Tracking Worksheet

by Dr. Arthur H. Kebo

at

https://www.createspace.com/3865989

Save Money Checklist Worksheet – Volume 1

by Dr. Arthur H. Kebo

at

https://www.createspace.com/3865992

Save Money Checklist Worksheet – Volume 2

by Dr. Arthur H. Kebo

at

https://www.createspace.com/3865993

www.ingramcontent.com/pod-product-compliance
Lightning Source LLC
Chambersburg PA
CBHW060006300526
45794CB00003B/1114